ZAHARIA TUDOREL

PATIENT CARE WITH ANOREXIA

NURSING

BUCHAREST 2024

Table of Contents

INTRODUCTION

Anorexia nervosa is an eating disorder characterized by an abnormally low body weight, an intense fear of gaining weight, and a distorted perception of weight . Symptoms of anorexia include extreme weight loss, thin appearance, abnormal blood counts, fatigue, insomnia, dizziness or fainting, bluish discoloration of the fingers, hair that thins, breaks or falls out, soft, downy hair covering the body, absence of menstruation, constipation, dry or yellowish skin, intolerance of cold, irregular heart rhythms, low blood pressure, dehydration, osteoporosis, swelling of arms or legs, and more . Patients with anorexia nervosa require specialized care from a team of medical professionals, including a medical doctor, a registered dietitian nutritionist, a psychotherapist, and a psychiatrist . The role of nurses is critical in identifying destructive eating patterns and providing physical and emotional care for patients from detection to recovery .

Anatomy and physiology of the digestive system

The digestive tract is made up of the following segments: mouth, pharynx (with double membership), esophagus, stomach, small intestine and large intestine.

The mouth is the initial portion of the digestive system, made up of organs and various tissues. Superiorly it is limited by the palatine vault, inferiorly by the floor of the mouth, laterally by the cheeks, anteriorly by the lips and posteriorly it continues with the pharynx. The oral cavity is lined with oral mucosa.

In the oral cavity there are the two dental arches, upper and lower, located on the maxilla and, respectively, on the mandible.
There are 32 teeth: 8 incisors, 4 canines, 8 premolars and 12 molars.
The tongue, a muscular organ located posteriorly,

presents on its upper surface some small shapes called papillae: filiform, fungiform and circumvallate or gustatory, the latter being located towards the root of the tongue and forming the lingual "V". In the oral cavity, the salivary, parotid, submaxillary and sublingual glands excrete saliva.

The functions performed by the mouth are: the function of mastication for the formation of the food bowl, the beginning of the digestion of carbohydrates under the action of the salivary gland, the function of phonation, the function of reception, the function of defense and the physiognomic function.

The pharynx is an organ that belongs to both the digestive system and the respiratory system. It is located in the posterior part of the oral cavity and continues with the esophagus. Lined with a mucous membrane, it is rich in lymphoid tissue. In the pharynx there are the palatine tonsils, the pharyngeal tonsil on the posterior wall and the lingual tonsil at the root of the tongue, connected to each other by numerous lymphatic vessels and forming the Waldeyer lymphatic ring.

The functions of the pharynx are: the function of leading the food bowl to the esophagus and the function of defense against infections, which can enter through the digestive or respiratory tract.

The esophagus is a muscular-membranous, tubular organ that connects the pharynx and the stomach. It starts at the level of the 7th cervical vertebra (C7) near the cricoid cartilage, and ends near the 11th thoracic vertebra at the cardia; it is 25 - 32 cm long and has a caliber that varies between 10 and 22 mm. It has three physiological straits: the cricoid strait, the strait at the level of the crossing with the aorta artery and the one at the level of the cardia. The esophagus is located in the posterior mediastinum, coming into contact with the formations located here. Because of this situation, the affections of the esophagus can spread to the organs with which it comes into contact, and on the other hand, their injuries can cause esophageal suffering. As a structure, the esophagus is made up of three layers: inside is the mucosa, with a stratified squamous epithelium; follows the middle tunic, which is muscular and has two layers - an internal one with circular fibers and an external one, with longitudinal fibers ; the tunica externa is made up of loose connective tissue, which continues with the mediastinal supporting tissue.

Physiologically, the esophagus is an organ meant to connect the pharynx and the stomach. Through the swallowing reflex, the food bowl passes from the pharynx to the esophagus; through nervous coordination, the muscles form contraction waves that push the bolus towards the cardia; the sphincter of the cardia opens, preventing the reflux of gastric contents into the esophagus. The existence of two anatomical areas with sphincter activity is accepted: one located at the pharyngo-esophageal junction and another, in the vicinity of the hiatal ring, at the border between the esophagus proper and the gastro-esophageal vestibule.

The stomach, a muscular-glandular cavity organ, is the segment of the digestive tube located between the esophagus and the small intestine. Its shape is similar to that of a pear, with the tip slightly bent and pointing upwards: in the radiology exam it appears like the letter "J" or like a hook. Its shape is variable depending on: content, the tonicity of the own muscles, the tonicity of the abdominal wall, the position of the individual and the volume of the neighboring organs.

The stomach starts from the cardia, which connects the esophagus and the stomach; the portion located above the cardia and which is adapted to the diaphragmatic dome, is called *the great tuberosity (fomix* or *fundus);* the vertical segment is *the body of the stomach,* which continues with *the small tuberosity* and then with *the pyloric antrum* and ends with *the pyloric orifice.*

between the cardia and the pylorus there are two edges: the external edge or *the great curvature* and the internal edge or *the small curvature.*

Structurally, the stomach is made up of four layers: on the inside is the mucosa, then submucosa, muscular, and on the outside it is covered by the peritoneal serosa. The mucosa is made up of a cylindrical epithelium, which secretes mucus, and the glands of the stomach: *the fundic glands, which* secrete hydrochloric acid and pepsin, *the pyloric glands* and *muciparous cells,* both of which secrete mucus. The muscle consists of an internal layer with obliquely arranged fibers, an intermediate layer with circular fibers and an external layer with longitudinal fibers. The circular layer, at the level of the pylorus, is very strong, constituting *the pyloric sphincter.*

From a physiological point of view , the stomach receives food and, thanks to its motor function, kneads it, mixes it with gastric juice and then evacuates it into the duodenum. Through the secretory function, the stomach intervenes in the digestion of connective tissue and proteins with the help of hydrochloric acid and pepsi ne. The gastric mucus has a first-order protective role, protecting the mucosa from the action of the gastric juice.

Gastric secretion is triggered first by a reflex-nervous mechanism, then by neuro-chemical mechanisms starting in the gastric mucosa *(gastric phase,* with gastrin secretion) and the small intestine *(intestinal phase).*

The small intestine begins at the pylorus and ends at the level of the ileo-cecal valve. It has three segments: duodenum, jejunum and ileum. *The duodenum* is shaped like a horseshoe. Four portions are described: *the first portion, the duodenal bulb,* follows immediately after the pylorus and is slightly mobile; *the second portion,* the descent, is located to the right of the spine and into it the biliary and pancreatic secretions are poured; **the third portion** is horizontal, **and the fourth portion** is ascending and continues with the jejunum, forming **the duodeno-jejunal angle.** Structurally, the duodenum is made up of four layers: mucosa, submucosa, muscular (with circular and longitudinal muscle fibers) and peritoneal serosa, which covers it only on the front side.

Physiologically, the duodenum has two main functions: motor and secretory. Duodenal motility pushes food chyme very quickly into the jejunum (in a few seconds). The duodenal secretion produces **secretin** (with a role in stimulating the pancreas and intestine), **enterokinase** (which transforms trypsinogen into trypsin) and **mucus.** At the level of the duodenum, the alimentary chyme arriving from the stomach begins to mix with duodenal juice, bile and pancreatic juice.

The jejuno-ileum has a smaller caliber and fills most of the peritoneal cavity. It is also made up of four layers:

mucosa, submucosa, muscular and serous. Unlike the duodenum, the serosa covers the entire circumference of the jejuno-ileum.

The mucosa forms circular folds *(convulsive valves)* and countless *intestinal villi,* creating an enormous surface, with a great role in intestinal absorption. In the terminal portion of the ileum, there are numerous lymphatic follicles, forming Payer's plates.

Physiologically, the jejuno-ileum has three functions: motor, secretory and absorption. The motor function is represented by *the pendular movements,* with the role of kneading and mixing the intestinal contents, and *by the peristaltic movements,* with the role of propelling the intestinal chyme. The secretory function is manifested by the production of enzymes: *erepsin* and *nucleotidase,* with a role in the digestion of proteins and nucleic acids; *intestinal lipase,* with a role in splitting neutral fats; *disaccharides* [maltase, isomaltase, sucrase (invertase), lactase], with a role in digesting carbohydrates to monosaccharides.

The absorption function is performed on a very large surface, thanks to the intestinal villi. Together with the aforementioned food principles, water, mineral salts and vitamins are also absorbed.

The large intestine is the terminal segment of the digestive tube; it starts from the ileo-cecal valve and ends with ***the anus.*** It is distinguished from the small intestine by its much larger volume and by the three longitudinal muscular bands (***taenia coli).*** Its length varies between 1.5 and 3 meters. The large intestine is divided into the following segments: cecum, ascending colon, transverse colon, descending colon, sigmoid colon and rectum.

The check is located in the right iliac fossa; the connection between the ileum and the cecum is made through ***the ileo-cecal sphincter*** (muscular formation).

On the inside of the check is *the appendix,* whose position is variable. The check has a degree of mobility.

The ascending colon is located on the right flank and continues the cecum, ascending vertically to the lower face of the liver, where, through the hepatic angle (right angle), it
continues with *the transverse colon.* It is fixed to the posterior wall of the abdomen through the peritoneum.

The transverse colon extends from the hepatic angle to the splenic angle (a left colon) and is located horizontally or in the shape of the letter "V".

The descending colon is located in the left flank and extends from the splenic angle to the level of the iliac crest, where it continues through the sigmoid colon.
The sigmoid colon, continuing the previous one, located in the left iliac fossa and in the pelvis, has the shape of an "S" and extends to the recto-sigmoid angle.

The rectum is the terminal portion: it extends from the recto-sigmoid angle to the anus and is located in the pelvis. The rectum communicates with the outside through the anal canal, which continues the rectal ampulla.

Structurally, the large intestine is made up of four layers: mucosa, submucosa, muscular and serous. The mucosa is very rich in mucous cells: the muscularis is characterized by the three longitudinal muscle bands and the transverse bands, which make up the haustra of the large intestine.

Physiologically, the large intestine has motility, secretion and absorption functions. Motility ensures the progression of the fecal bolus through peristaltic, segmental contractions, and through massive contractions. The faecal bowl collects in the sigmoid; the passage of fecal matter into the rectum leads to their expulsion through the physiological act of defecation.

The secretion of the large intestine is reduced to mucus.

The absorption function is reduced and is exercised, especially, at the level of the check and the ascendant; water, salts, vitamins, glucose are absorbed. At the level of the rectum, medicinal substances and water can be absorbed , reaching the inferior vena cava.

1. Introduction

Anorexia nervosa is a psychiatric disorder in the category of eating disorders, characterized by an abnormal reduction in body weight and a distortion of the perception of one's own body image with a prevalent, persistent fear of gaining weight.
People suffering from anorexia nervosa limit their body weight by voluntarily abstaining from food for a long time.

The first clinical observations of anorexic patients were made by Richard Morton at the end of the 17th century (1694). It was only in 1873 that the London doctor William Gull and the neuropsychiatrist Ernest Lasseque independently published descriptions of the disease, considering it to be a disorder on the spectrum of hysteria - "hysterical anorexia"

In 1883 H. Huchard called it anorexia nervosa

In 1950 Hilde Bruch observed that this abnormal behavior was aimed at losing weight "the only success in the unhappy world in which these girls lived".

2. Definition

Anorexia nervosa is characterized by self-imposed starvation and the refusal to keep the weight at a minimal value corresponding to the age and height associated with an intense fear of not gaining weight. These eating disorders characteristic of teenagers are characterized by:

- the morbid perception regarding the weight and shape of the body

- severe disturbance of eating behavior

Epidemiological aspects

In anorexia nervosa, the average age is 15-17 years.

Psychogenic anorexic behavior can be found from the first week of life, in infants but also in early childhood, the prevalence in psychiatric hospitals being 1-5%

In general, the prevalence of anorexia nervosa in general in the female population throughout life is estimated at 0.1 - 0.7%

The studies conducted found a prevalence rate of anorexia nervosa of 0.5-1% in women in the last part of adolescence and the beginning of the adult period.

There are few data regarding the male sex.

Although most teenage girls make efforts to be thin, anorexia develops only in those who show certain personality traits. Obsessive-compulsive traits, perfectionism, rigidity, narcissistic and hysterical traits, immaturity and fear of assuming responsibilities were also frequently cited.

The mortality rate in eating disorders is 10%.

The most common cause of death is starvation, cardiac disorders (due to electrolyte imbalances) or suicide.

3. Etiopathogenesis

Eating behavior disorders have a multifactorial etiology. The factors involved in their etiopathogenesis can be grouped into: genetic, socio-cultural and psychological.

a) **Genetic factors** are involved in eating behavior disorders, a fact demonstrated by recent controlled family studies that showed an increased prevalence throughout life in first-degree relatives of patients with anorexia nervosa: 3-12%, compared to the groups control – 0-3.7%.

In anorexia nervosa in first degree relatives of individuals with anorexia nervosa. Thus, daughters of patients with anorexia nervosa have a 6.6% risk of developing anorexia nervosa.

It was also found that individuals with eating disorders have a high level of vasopressin and cortisol.

Both hormones are involved in the body's response to physical and emotional stress.

Other studies have found increased levels of neuropeptide-Y and peptide YY in patients with anorexia nervosa, suggesting that they may play a role in eating behavior disorders.

b) **Psychological factors** - Psychoanalytic theories explain eating behavior disorders through the existence of a seductive, dependent relationship of the adolescent towards the passive, warm, but lacking in authority father figure and a sense of guilt sustained by an obsessive anorexia nervosa, bivalent anorexia nervosa, with which the teenager refuses to identify.

Some studies have shown that perfectionism is associated in these patients with rituals related to food and with a greater resistance to change regarding food behavior.

In the case of anorexia nervosa behavior in infants and small children, it seems that it would be due to inappropriate attitudes of the mother with the disruption of the mother-child relationship, which downgrades anorexia from opposition, the child thus confronting the mother, who becomes either hyperanxious, rejecting and rigid. Other factors involved may be child abuse and neglect. The apparent control over eating behavior, restrictive diets seem to provide a false self-control in everyday life in patients with anorexia nervosa.

c) **Socio-cultural factors** - The inability to recognize and react correctly to the needs of the body - such as the feeling of hunger associated with the need to reach the beauty standards imposed by contemporary society and constantly promoted by the media channels are just some of the etiopathogenic hypotheses regarding eating disorders.

4. Symptomatology

Anorexia nervosa begins especially during puberty and adolescence, in young girls with a solid education, who live in an environment of extreme dependence, obedient and studious with very good school results, perfectionists with episodes of early anorexia nervosa, dietary whims and illnesses in the antecedents.

Forms of anorexia nervosa:

- in infants:

an anorexia of inertia - the child does not swallow

oppositional anorexia - restlessness, food rejection, vomiting .

- in preschoolers: as a reaction of opposition to the rigidity of the parents who impose quantitative and qualitative food excesses, strict meal times, whims in the choice of food.

- in adolescence: food restrictions can appear as a result of an emotional shock or psychological conflicts, sometimes they gradually set in without an apparent cause, as a result of a weight loss regime or conflicting situations that the adolescent cannot resolve.

There are two types of anorexia nervosa:

- the restrictive type

- the type of excessive eating/purging

Binge eating/purging type : this type is used when the adolescent engaged in regular binge eating or purging or both during the current episode. The adolescent with anorexia nervosa who eats excessively purges herself through self-induced vomiting or abuse of diuretics, laxatives or enemas. At other times he does not eat excessively, but regularly purges after consuming small amounts of food.

The restrictive type describes the clinical picture in which weight loss is achieved primarily through diet, fasting or excessive physical exercise. Over time, disorders appear secondary to the decrease in food intake: bones are visible under the dry skin, sparse and brittle hair, cold and cyanotic extremities, loose tongue, constipation.

The clinical aspect in anorexia nervosa is very particular, the symptoms can appear after an event perceived as psychotraumatizing or most often after malicious remarks about the weight of the patients.

Teenage girls with the intention of losing weight engage in drastic diets.

Avoid eating carbohydrates and fats, which is why I exclude them from the diet. They are subject to a regime of self-information. Afterwards, they no longer recognize the feeling of hunger. They frequently control their weight, they rigorously compose their diet, so that the number of calories ingested is reduced, most of the time below 500 cal/day (they end up eating only one apple a day or fasting). Some patients resort to true rituals regarding eating behavior, for example, small amounts of food are cut into very small pieces to be eaten or they set the table in a certain way.

5. Characteristics

a) Behavioral characteristics

☐Most of the time, anorexia nervosa is triggered by a particular psychotraumatic event: they feel rejected, they are vulnerable, sometimes they start a weight loss regime. Events such as separation from parents, school difficulties, the ironies of the entourage can intervene.

b) Affective characteristics

☐Losing weight is for them a sign of power that allows them to dominate their surroundings. Anorexics are often people ruled by fear: fear of becoming an adult and expressing responsibilities, fear of losing control over food.

c) Cognitive characteristics

☐Anorexics have the desire to lose weight and to maintain control over their diet corresponds to an egosynthotic behavior - that is, a behavior that agrees with their own ideas, desires and values (denies hunger, physical and mental exhaustion). For them, the obsession with food is a normal behavior.

d) Socio-cultural characteristics

In a study done in 1982, it was considered that 70-80% of female students do not consider themselves seductive because they are not thin due to the existence of the fashion of being thin=mannequin.

In American society, the figure is generally synonymous with seduction.

It was found that eating disorders are frequent in middle to upper societies (Russel 1985, Butler 1988); high incidence among young women from wealthy families

6. Paraclinical and laboratory data

Individuals with anorexia nervosa do not show laboratory abnormalities, this disorder can affect most major systems and organs and produces a variety of disturbances.

The abnormalities are transient, inconstant and reversible upon weight gain.

Heart rate is slower, EKG changes occur.

Hematological changes: marked anemia, increased blood urea, reversible abnormalities unrelated to weight loss, and the immune system remains surprisingly effective.

Endocrinological changes: related to the disruption of the hypothalamic-pituitary axis:

- global depression of pituitary-ovarian activity

- secretion of LH (luteinizing hormone) similar to prepubescent fetuses

- disruption of estrogen metabolism

- EEG shows diffuse abnormalities, reflects metabolic encephalopathy, can result from significant changes in fluids and electrolytes.

Energy expenditure for relaxation is relatively low.

7. Positive diagnosis

DSM diagnostic criteria for anorexia nervosa.

A) Refusal to maintain a normal body weight or above one

minimum normal weights for his age and height.

B) Intense fear of not gaining weight or becoming fat

C) Disturbance of the way weight or body shape is expressed not due to the influence of weight or body shape.

D) In postmenarcheal women, amenorrhea occurs - the absence of at least 3 consecutive menstrual cycles.

We specify the type:

- type of excessive eating, the person regularly engages in excessive eating behavior
- restrictive type, the person does not regularly engage in purging behavior.

8. Differential diagnosis

The differential diagnosis is the same as the characterized superior mesenteric artery syndrome. through postprandial vomiting following pylorus obstruction.

The differential diagnosis will concern the mental disorders in which anorexia-like symptoms such as:

• Major depressive disorder. in which the patient can lose weight, as a result of the decrease in appetite, but unlike anorexia nervosa, he is not concerned about diet or body shape, he does not have an excessive fear of not gaining weight. However, anorexia nervosa can be associated with a depressive syndrome characterized by depressed mood and low self-esteem. affective lability.

• Schizophrenia, in which the patient may exhibit bizarre behavior related to food, possibly with weight loss but without being concerned about his image.

• Obsessive-convulsive disorder, patients with anorexia nervosa can have obsessions and convulsions but only in connection with eating behavior.

• Social phobia: patients may have an avoidance behavior, but this is only related to eating behavior.

• Body dysmorphic disorder: the patient is concerned not only with body weight but also with other imaginary defects of it.

- Food negativism, schizophrenia

- Negative catatonic psychosis

- Hysterical anorexia

- Obsessive anorexia accompanied by food rituals

- Food phobia is often accompanied by other phobias and/or obsessions

9. Evolution, prognosis

They are variable in anorexia nervosa, there can be a complete recovery after a single episode, but most often the evolution is fluctuating with exacerbations and partial remissions.

The evolution of infants and children is generally favorable with the improvement of this behavior over time.

In anorexia nervosa, the favorable prognostic factors are: age under 18, lack of previous hospitalizations, absence of purging behavior.

The unfavorable ones are: intra-family conflicts, associated personality disorders.

10. Evaluation methods

Patients with anorexia nervosa resist consultation, so it is important to establish a good relationship.

The detailed history of the development of the disorder, data on the current diet, weight control and the patient's ideas about the corporate weight are taken into consideration.

Three types of eating disorder assessment tools are developed:

A. observation conversation

B. observation scales

C. self-questionnaires

The observation conversation

- the standardized observation guide according to ASM III, DSM III R and ICD 10 which contain lists of precise questions for anorexia nervosa

- DIS (Diagnostic Interview Schedule, Robrius. 1985);

- SCAN (Schedule for Clinical Assessment in Neuropsychiatry, Wing, (1988)

- CIDI (Composite International Diagnostic Interview, WHO 1981)

- SCID (Structured Clinical Interview for DSM IIIR, Spitzer &Co, 1988)

Observation scales: for evaluating the severity of anorexic behaviors during supervision and monitoring their evolution.

- Slade's scale (Anorexic Behavior Scale, 1973)

- EBRS (Eating Behavior Rating Scale. Wilson & Co)

C) <u>Self-questionnaire</u> : for the common assessment of clients with eating disorders:

- EAT (Eating Attitudes Test, Garfiedul & Garner, 1979) most often used, provides a confirmation of the diagnosis.

- EDI (Eating Disorder Inventatiry, Gamer & Co, 1983) includes 64 positions for evaluating the subject's physical and behavioral traits

11. Treatment

In anorexia nervosa in adolescents, treatment is difficult due to the fact that patients with anorexia nervosa are ambivalent about treatment.

The treatment consists first of all in obtaining an adequate weight.

For this purpose, a rigorous food plan will be developed together with the patient. Thus, the target weight and weight gain rate per week will be negotiated with him, the calories needed to reach this target will be calculated, the diet will be established according to the foods that the patient accepts and divided into 5 meals a day, 3 main meals and 2 snacks that contain all the nutritional principles: proteins, carbohydrates, lipids, vitamins, minerals.The patient can be treated in an outpatient setting or in a hospital.

Psychotherapeutic treatment involves supportive, cognitive-behavioral, family therapy with the establishment of a solid therapeutic relationship between patient and psychiatrist.

The psychopharmacological treatment consists in the administration of tricyclic antidepressants, selective serotonin reuptake inhibitors that have proven effective in the hospital when there are depressive symptoms or associated obsessive-phobic behaviors.

INDIVIDUAL PSYCHOTHERAPY:
The therapist directs his attention to the dynamic meaning of the affection; the preoccupation with food and weight masks fundamental problems and numerous doubts.

In general, the anorexic patient refuses to talk and/or acknowledge his illness and avoids collaboration with the therapist. The therapist must earn his trust and motivate him to change his behavior. It helps him to have confidence in his own strengths, to make decisions even if sometimes they are hasty and to accept new forms of adaptation to stressful situations. The beneficial effects of the treatment must be emphasized with the assurance that it will not affect the goal proposed by the patient (maintaining the silhouette)Cognitive-behavioral therapy aims to identify and modify erroneous perceptions regarding food, weight and body shape on self-esteem.

GROUP PSYCHOTHERAPY: teenagers in homogenous groups look for their roles, comment on behaviors in comparison with behavioral standards.

FAMILY PSYCHOTHERAPY

according to some clinicians, family separation is a vital feature of the treatment, and according to others, on the contrary, it has a key role in the rehabilitation of the anorexic.

The therapy is focused on both the eating and emotional problems of the adolescent.

MEDICINE THERAPY

In drug therapy, successes have been reported with tranquilizers, sedative and incisive neuroleptics that make the patient less afraid of weight gain.Research was done on the effect of Fluoxetine compared to that of the placebo group, as a result of which it was found that the opportunity to administer Fluoxetine is limited.

12. Conclusions

Anorexia expresses a crisis of development against the background of a vulnerable personality that appeared at puberty or in adolescence, characterized by deliberate weight loss, loss induced and sustained by the patient. Weight loss is achieved by eliminating the amount of ingested food.Anorexia nervosa seems to result from the combination of an individual predisposition and factors of any nature that encourage dieting. Once the disorder is established, the family's response can favor its perpetuation.Anorexia nervosa is considered a psychological disorder requiring immediate intervention to restore body weight, remove anxiety and restore interpersonal relationships.The self-esteem of individuals with anorexia nervosa is extremely dependent on their body weight and shape.

Special care given to hospitalized patients

- Hospitalization of the patient

Hospitalization is an important event in the patient's life; he separates from his usual environment and is forced to resort to the help of strangers.

Hospitalization is based on referrals from the family doctor. Hospitalized patients are registered at the Reception Service Office in the admissions register, where the clinical observation sheet is also filled in with the patient's identity data.

The patients will be examined upon admission by the doctor on duty, who will collect the anamnestic data from the patient or companion and write them down in the observation sheet, establishing the necessary presumptive diagnosis from the point of view of directing the patient to the hospital wards. In view of the clinical examination, carried out by the doctor on duty, medical assistance helps the patient to undress.

After establishing the presumptive diagnosis and assigning the patient to the ward, medical assistance accompanies the patient to the bathroom, helps him undress, observes the integuments and fascia (if necessary, deworms the patient), helps him bathe (if he cannot), then leads to the dressing room where she helps him to put on his hospital clothes (pajamas, stockings, slippers, gown).

The patient's clothes will be taken over and registered carefully for storage, issuing a pick-up slip to the patient or the companion (if needed, the clothes will also be dewormed).

Thus prepared, the assistant leads the patient to the salon where he is introduced to the other patients, informs him about the hospital's internal order regulations and helps him sit in the bed prepared with clean linen.

After the patient has been put to bed, the medical assistance draws up the temperature sheet, determines the patient's weight, measures T0, pulse, BP, and records the obtained data in the observation sheet.

Medical assistance will also reassure the patient's family members, assuring them of the quality care that the patient will benefit from in the hospital, informing them of the number of the room where the patient was admitted and the schedule of visits.

Welcoming patients to the ward and introducing them to the customs of the ward is a decisive moment in gaining the patient's trust in the medical staff.

- Ensuring environmental conditions

Comfortable

The therapeutic protection regime aims to create hospitalization conditions that ensure patients maximum comfort, mental and physical well-being. Sections with beds, with what goes into their endowment: lounges, corridors, must have a pleasant appearance. The salon for the sick will fulfill, in addition to the hygiene requirements, the aesthetic and comfort requirements.

It is recommended to orient the hospital rooms to the southeast, south or southwest. The beds are separated, so that the patients do not disturb each other.

- ***Ventilation***

It is done by opening the windows in the morning after the patient goes to the toilet, after treatments, visits to the doctor, after meals, visitors and whenever necessary. Odorants will be sprayed for olfactory comfort.

Humidifying the air in the room, in a percentage of 55-60%, is absolutely mandatory, because an atmosphere that is too dry irritates the upper respiratory tract.

Natural lighting is ensured by wide windows, which must present at least ¼ of the living room area.

Heating is provided by central heating. The temperature is continuously controlled with room thermometers, in order to achieve: in the adults' rooms a temperature of 18-19 ºC and in the children's rooms 20-23 ºC.

Silence is another condition that must be ensured for hospitalized patients, because the patient can be easily irritated by noise. Sleep is a very important therapeutic factor, having to be deep and longer than usual.

- Ensuring hygiene

The patient's toilet is part of the basic care, i.e. the care provided by the medical assistant with the aim of ensuring the patient's comfort and hygiene.

It consists in maintaining the skin in a state of perfect cleanliness and in preventing the appearance of skin lesions, being an essential condition for healing.

The patient toilet can be:

- daily by region;

- weekly or general bathroom

Depending on the type of patient:

- does not need help;

- he needs physical and mental support;

- needs partial help;

- requires complete help.

Objectives:

● removal from the surface of the skin of the flaky corneous layer impregnated with the secretions of the sebaceous and sweat glands;

● the opening of the secretion holes of the skin glands;

● invigorating skin circulation and the whole body;

● the production of an active hyperemia of the skin, which favors the mobilization of antibodies;

● calming the patient, creating a pleasant state of comfort;

● the ambient temperature is checked, to avoid cooling the patient;

● avoid drafts by closing windows and doors

● the patient is isolated from his entourage;

- the materials necessary for the toilet, for changing the linen, for the bed and for the patient are prepared in order to prevent bedsores;

- the patient will be completely undressed and covered with a sheet and blanket;

- only the part to be washed is gradually revealed;

- squeeze the sponge or bath glove correctly, so that water does not leak into the bed or on the patient;

- soap and rinse with a firm hand, without brutality to promote blood circulation;

- warm water must be plentiful, changed as often as needed, without leaving the soap in the water;

- it is insisted on folds, under the breasts, on the hands and in the interdigital spaces, at the elbows and armpits

- the joints are immobilized in all their amplitude and the areas prone to pressure sores are massaged;

- the order in which the toilet is done by region: washed, rinsed, dried;

- move the mask and the protective cover depending on the region we are washing.

- Feeding the patient

The diet will be started only with liquid, then with a soft consistency so that it can be swallowed by the patient, who often has swallowing and mastication problems. Depending on the condition of the patient, his feeding is done:

- active

- passive

Passive nutrition

- the patient is placed in a semi-sitting position with the help of the bed rest or in supine position with the head slightly raised and bent forward to facilitate swallowing;

- his underwear is protected with a clean towel;

- arrange a towel around the neck;

- the table is adapted to the bed and the food is placed so that he can see what is put in his mouth;

- assistance sits to the right of the patient and gently raises his head with a pillow;

- check the temperature of the food;

- serves him soup with a spoon or from a cup with a beak, cuts solid foods;

- supervises the liquid flow to avoid overloading the patient's swallowing capacity;

- his mouth is wiped, his bed is made;

- remove possible feeding residues that have reached under the patient and may contribute to possible bedsores;

- covers the patient and ventilates the room;

- Preparing the patient for explorations

-Psychological preparation of the patient:

The attitude towards the patient must reflect the permanent desire to help him; creating a favorable climate; the close attitude constitutes the important factors of a good mental preparation.

In the vicinity of examinations of any nature, medical assistance must clarify the patient on the harmless nature of the examinations, seeking to minimize pain.

The patient must never be misled, because otherwise he will lose his trust in us.

Undressing and dressing the patient:

The patient should not be completely naked in front of any examination, but the partial uncovering of the surfaces to be examined by pulling and twisting the shirt around the patient's neck should not be practiced, as this can hide a number of important symptoms.

After the clinical examination, the patient must be dressed in hospital clothes. Dressing and undressing must be done very tactfully and delicately so as not to cause pain.

- Patient supervision

- assistance will visit the patient as often as possible, even without request;

- will follow and note the pathological manifestations such as: hemorrhages, behavioral manifestations, contractions or convulsions and will report them to the doctor;

- will note volumetric liquid eliminations;

-assistance will determine the density of each urine emission and note it in the FO;

- you will follow TA, P, R, T°, and in cases of constipation he will do an evacuation enema.

- Administration of treatment

The administration of the treatment is done respecting the hygiene conditions, the dose recommended by the doctor and the schedule. For a light administration, the intravenous route is used with the help of a needle, which saves the patient from multiple stings. Also, medical assistance will educate the patient to avoid self-medication.

Monitoring of vital and vegetative functions

a. P pulse

It can be taken on any palpable artery that can be compressed on a bony plane (radial, temporal, carotid, femoral, humeral, posterior pedicle).

The patient will be at physical and mental rest for 10-15 minutes before the count. The radial groove is noted at the distal extremity of the forearm in continuation of the police.

Palpation of the pulse is done with the tip of the index, middle and ring fingers of the right hand. A slight pressure is applied on the arterial wall with the three fingers until the full pulse beats are felt. The fixation of the fingers is done with the help of the police that embraces the forearm at the respective level. The counting is done for one minute with the help of a second hand clock.

The notation in the temperature sheet is done

with a red pen, counting four pulsations for each horizontal line.

Normal values for adults are between 60-80 pulses/minute.

b. Blood pressure

For blood pressure measurement, the patient will be physically and mentally prepared.

The cuff is applied supported and in extension with the arm, the membrane of the stethoscope is fixed on the humeral artery under the inner edge of the cuff. The olives of the stethoscope are inserted into the ears, air is pumped into the pneumatic cuff with the help of the rubber pair until the pulsating noises disappear. The air in the cuff is progressively decompressed by opening the valve until the first arterial sound is perceived, which represents the maximum blood pressure value. The value indicated by the mercury column or the manometer needle is retained to be recorded. The decompression continues, the arterial noises becoming stronger, the value indicated by the mercury column or the manometer needle is retained at the moment the noises disappear, this value representing the minimum arterial pressure.

The obtained values are noted in the temperature sheet with a red horizontal line, counting for each line of the sheet one unit of the mercury column. Join the horizontal lines with vertical lines and hatch the resulting space.

Normal values for adults are: maximum blood pressure 115-140 mmHg and minimum blood pressure 75-90 mmHg.

c. Breathing

During the measurement of breathing, the patient will be placed in a supine position without explaining the technique to be performed with the palm of the hand on the palmar surface on the chest. Breaths are counted for one minute. Breathing can be assessed by simply observing the respiratory movements by lifting and the return of the chest to normal.

On the temperature sheet, note in green, each

horizontal line representing two breaths.

Normal values for adults: evening 20 breaths/minute, morning 18 breaths/minute.

d. D iuresis

To determine the amount of urine emitted in 24 hours, the patient will be instructed to urinate only in the urinal for 24 hours. The graduated cylindrical vessels will be well covered and kept cool to prevent fermentation processes.

Along with recording the diuresis value, the amount of fluids ingested will also be recorded. The ratio between the amount of fluids ingested and those eliminated reflects the balance of water circulation in the body.The normal value is around 1500 ml/24 hours. In men it is 1200-1800 ml/24 hours, in women 1000-1400 ml/24 hours.

Patient discharge

For the specialist medical assistant, the patient's discharge from the hospital must be a concern, as it was shown that his reception must be.

A large segment of patients do not raise problems at discharge, they know the date of discharge, they can move on their own but with difficulty due to paresis of different parts of the body.

In these situations, the specialist medical assistant must take care that the discharge forms carried out by the doctor reach the patients on time, give some additional clarifications, if the patient did not perfectly understand the clarifications given and written by the doctor and, by his attitude, to show the patient the concern he has for him until the moment he leaves the hospital.

CHAPTER II. CASE STUDY

Case 1.

Introduction

The attention given to the patient is very important, taking into account the fact that the patient who requests medical care puts his life and health in the hands of the care staff. This trust implies responsibilities but also many qualities: kindness, politeness, generosity, tact and professionalism.

The nurse contributes to activities involved in the care of the mentally ill that sometimes seem simple, but they must be individualized, adapted to the needs and possibilities of each patient.

The role of the nurse, said Virginia Henderson - the promoter of the concept of nursing, is to help the individual, whether sick or healthy, to find their way to health or rehabilitation, to use their every action to promote health.

In patient care, the nurse participates in data collection activities, identification of care problems, establishment of long-term and short-term objectives, implementation of the care plan and evaluation.

1. Data collection: the interview with the patient, the family, data obtained from other professionals.

2. Identifying care problems consists in classifying ideas and establishing possibilities.

3. Establishing long-term and short-term objectives: the purpose and planning of preferred care together with the patient and her family.

4. Implementation of the care plan: organization of actual care activities, planning interventions in relation to the needs of the individual.

5. Evaluation: analysis of the results obtained from the patient.

B) Presentation of the case

"FRA CARITATIS" TRAINING CENTER

OBSERVATION SHEET FOR PSYCHIATRIC NURSING

I. Anamnestic data

Name, Surname – MS

Marital status - unmarried

Date of birth – 10.09.1994

Current occupation - student

Address, Telephone – District.Maramures , Bodes Township

Studies - 8th grade, General School no. 1

Allergies - food

II. self help	Independent	Need help	addicted
1. Mobility	Yes	-	-
2. Feeding	-	Yes	-
3. Hygiene	Yes	-	-
4. Dressed	Yes	-	-
5. The continent	Yes	-	-

III. Patient description

a) Eye color: blue

b) Hair color: satin

c) Height: 1.54 m

d) Weight: 40 kg

e) Skin: white

f) Teeth: complete dentition, shows two caries

g) Vision: good

h) Manners: does not present

i) Speech: coherence

j) Physical deformities/posture: none

2. The patient's preferred name: Miky

3. Distinctive features

4. Previous occupation: student

5. Hobbies and interests: reading, listening to music, hanging out with friends

6. Family members or significant persons in the patient's life: maternal grandparents, maternal aunt and mother.

7. People who could visit him / Social support: grandparents, aunt (the patient is hospitalized with her mother.

8. Living conditions: she lives in a two-room apartment with her maternal grandparents, maternal aunt and mother (46 years old, no longer working for medical reasons, parents are divorced, the patient does not keep in touch with her father, whom she only knows from view.)

IV. Mental condition

1	Previous mental illnesses: The patient was hospitalized in the pediatric hospital in Pitesti with the diagnosis of anorexia nervosa, the patient lost 21 kg in 2 months.	
2	Current mental state:	
	a)	General appearance: neat appearance, depressed face, easy crying, uncooperativeness, irritability
	b	Behavior: denies the existence of problems, low

	)	tolerance for frustration
c)		Communication (speech/content): verbal contact is established with difficulty, but the patient states that she gets along well with other colleagues.
		Nonverbal: visual contact is easily made but not maintained, the gaze is directed downwards
	d)	Mood: isolated, withdrawn, sad mood
	e)	Orientation: temporal-spatial
	f)	Sleep: physiological
	d)	How the patient understands his illness: he denies the existence of some problems
	h)	The family's attitude towards the patient's illness: the patient is cared for by her grandmother who accompanies her, the mother is very worried about the girl's condition, she said that "she doesn't know what else to do to

| | make her daughter feel better" |
| 3. Subjects of concern for the patient: |
| - food refusal |
| - obsessive preoccupation with weight |
| - severe weight loss |

V. Additional information:

The patient, aged 15 years and 7 months, student in the 8th grade, is hospitalized in the 5th ward of the Pr. Dr. Alexandru Obregia Hospital for:

- food refusal

- obsessive preoccupation with body weight

- distorted body image

The patient was hospitalized in the last two months in the Pediatric Hospital in Drobeta Turnu Severin with the diagnosis of anorexia nervosa, severe malnutrition following food refusal, from where she was transferred to our clinic for the establishment of therapeutic behavior.

The patient comes accompanied by her grandmother to our ward for the reappearance of exaggerated weight concerns.

The patient associates the onset of symptoms with the critical statement from a colleague "she told me that I am fat and ugly and I need to lose weight"

The patient's parents are divorced, the patient does not keep in touch with her father, whom she only knows by sight.

Other data

Laboratory data

GLU – 78 mg/dl

TP – 6.1 g/dl

CA – 8.0 mg/dl

AST – 20 U/L

ALT – 19 U/L

Ca $^{2+}$ - 1.80 MEg/L

Thymol – 1UML

HGB – 13.9 g/dL

L – 10.9 10^{6}/μL

H – 4.5 10^6/μL

Hz – 37.8%

T – 26.1 10^3/μL

EEG:

The EEG trace with diffuse bioelectric changes and voltage with tendencies to flatten the background trace. Hyperventilation does not significantly change the long-distance route; without paroxysmal discharges.

Psychological examination:

Anxious experiences related to the possibility of getting fat, distorted image of the silhouette, intense preoccupations to lose weight, relational inadequacy, the accentuated need to receive affection, over-appreciation, self-idealization, act in an orderly, methodical manner.

It shows restlessness, instability, irritability.

Under treatment with Olanzapine 15mg/day; Thioridazine 150 mg/day; Zoloft 100 mg/day; polyvitamins 2 tb/ day; 6 Glubifer 3 tb/day, the clinical evolution is satisfactory.

He is discharged at the request of the family with the recommendation to continue the treatment.

C. Data analysis and interpretation

Anorexia is a very serious eating behavior disorder, without treatment it leads to the emergence of not easy complications and even death.

The nurse must be patient with the patient, understanding, calm and firm with the patient. She must give the patient and the family as many details as possible about the disease and its treatment.

Basically, anorexics refuse to admit that they have a disorder and oppose any intervention aimed at their eating behavior, but at the same time they can more easily accept help to solve other problems.

The nurse, together with the patient and his family, will draw up the care plan, establish the schedule and content of the meals, taking into account the patient's food preferences, and will use different therapy techniques.

In family therapy, the nurse has the role of:

- helps the family to express their needs

- helps the patient to modify and control her answers

- discuss difficult problems in the family

- actively participates in finding solutions without imposing a certain option.

D. CARE PLAN

PURPOSE – LONG TERM

Date	No. Fr.	Identified needs/problems (Dr. Nursing)	Desired result (goal - short term)	Interventions (Actions/Date/Time)	Signature	Result obtained
07. 05. 09	1	Nutritional deficit, related to self-deprivation of food and hyperactivity	The patient will restore her normal body weight	- I established together with the patient and her grandmother the schedule and organization of meals, 4 small portions per day. - I went with the patient to the		

				dining room, where she ate with all the other patients in my presence. - I supervised the patient during and after the meal to avoid the provocation of vomiting and not to throw away the food. - I congratulated the patient when she managed to eat everything we proposed - I talked with the grandmother saying that a visible progress was obtained in terms of nutrition		

				and body weight		
				- I weighed the patient daily, in the morning in the same outfit.		
				- I tried by distracting the patient after each meal to make the patient stop crying by training her in different games in the playroom (card game, stick game)		
	2	Disturbance of self-esteem associated with a low tolerance	The patient will show an increase in self-	- I encouraged her to define her own interests (preferred activities) to make her feel less disinterested by gaining control		

		e to frustrati on, related to the need to please others, to be approve d, accepte d	estee m, she will gain more confid ence in her own strengt h	over herself - I talked with the patient about what she likes to do, how she would like to be in relationships with her parents and others and how acceptance will be achieved. - I strengthened the patient's strengths, valued her by making her more confident in her own strengths		
	3	Social isolation , disruptio n of interper	The patient will relate more easily	- I helped the patient talk about her feelings of loneliness through permanent		

		sonal relationships due to the fear of being rejected.	to others and participate in group activities or other social activities	interactions with her several times a day. - I showed a sincere interest to the patient, trying to convince her that I care about her - I encourage the patient to look for ways to spend her free time, to be able to relax, to broaden her social contacts. - I recommended the patient to avoid conflicts of any kind both with her grandmother and with her colleagues		

				through tolerance and self-confidence.		
	4	Anxiety about gaining weight and losing control over food	The patient will talk more easily about her fears	- I encouraged the patient to talk about her fears, implicitly about gaining weight and losing control over food. - through systematic discussions every day, I explained to the patient that there is progress in solving her major problems by gaining weight without distorting her image of her physique - I presented her		

| | | | | with a table showing the ideal weight for her age and height
- I discussed with the patient about the foods that do not pose a risk of making you fat, but on the contrary can be very beneficial in order to obtain a good functionality of the body (e.g. fruits, vegetables, dairy products) | | |
| | 5 | Disturba nce of family dynamic s due to rigidity | The family will becom e more unders | - I evaluated family relationships
- through discussions with the mother, | | |

| | | in the exercise of roles | tandin g, will be more open to the patient 's proble ms and will encour age her to act autono mously | different ways of approaching her relations with her daughter were suggested - from the dialogue with the patient's mother, she comes to the conclusion that she needs to reorganize her ideas and approach to situations. The patient will be controlled by the mother "from the shadows" without emphasizing the idea of eating out of obligation, thus de- escalating the | | |

				conflict between them - finally, the family is willing to adopt an open dialogue between them based on sincerity, which will help them have a harmonious relationship with the family.		

E. ASSESSMENT AND THE PATIENT'S RESPONSE TO CARE

Date	No. pb.		Signature
As a result of the care performed, the objectives were not achieved at all			
	1	The patient started to eat better, but the weight gain did not exceed 1 ½ during the 2-week hospitalization, still	

		maintaining control over the quality and quantity of food	
	2	The patient expressed her feelings referring to her own person and understood the functions and needs of the body	
		The patient has more self-confidence and has found ways to be accepted by others, showing tolerance and self-confidence	
		The patient wants to change her behavior, shows interest in the proposed activities and easily verbalizes her feelings.	
		The fear of not gaining weight has decreased in intensity, but it still persists.	
		The family showed understanding for the patient's problems in order to de-tension the situation in the family as much as possible, he will be permanently always by her side, without feeling constrained. Specifically, after the grandmother's departure from the hospital, the patient stayed with us for another week, during	

which she settled in better, was relaxed, more available in conversations, relating well with the salon colleagues with whom she ate together and played various games activities.

Under treatment with Olanzapine 15mg/day; Thioridazine 150 mg/day; Zoloft 100 mg/day; polyvitamins 2 tb/day; 6 Glubifer 3 tb/day, the clinical evolution is satisfactory.

He is discharged at the request of the family with the recommendation to continue the treatment.

F) Conclusions

Eating disorders (anorexia and bulimia nervosa) generally appear during puberty and adolescence against a background of increased psychological vulnerability, considering the increasingly demanding socio-cultural conditions, attention is directed towards the masses of young people to prevent the installation of these disorders.

For this, the care network in the community will have to be developed, the preparation of educational programs for teenagers, the development of relations with the educational institutions where the young people work. It is necessary to develop educational programs regarding eating disorders among young people, since they have a psychiatric and not an organic origin. It is desirable for the adolescent to know and understand his role in society.

Case 2

I. Anamnestic data

Name, Surname – CS

Marital status - unmarried

Current occupation - student

Address, Telephone –
District. Bucharest Township

Studies - 8th grade, General School no. 1

II. self help	Independent		addicted
1. Mobility	Yes	-	-
2. Feeding	-	Yes	-
3. Hygiene	Yes	-	-
4. Dressed	Yes	-	-
5. The continent	Yes	-	-

III. Patient description

a) Eye color: blue

b) Hair color: satin

c) Height: 1.64 m

d) Weight: 45 kg

e) Skin: white

f) Teeth: complete dentition, shows two caries

g) Vision: good

h) Manners: does not present

i) Speech: coherence

j) Physical deformities/posture: none

2. The patient's preferred name: Cathy

3. Distinctive features

4. Previous occupation: student

5. Hobbies and interests: reading, listening to music, hanging out with friends

6. Family members or significant persons in the patient's life: maternal grandparents, maternal aunt and mother.

7. People who could visit him / Social support: grandparents, aunt (the patient is hospitalized with her mother.

8. Living conditions: she lives in a two-room apartment with her maternal grandparents, maternal aunt and mother (46 years old, no longer working for medical reasons, parents are divorced, the patient does not keep in touch with her father, whom she only knows from view.)

IV. Mental condition

1	Previous mental illnesses: The patient was hospitalized in the pediatric hospital in Craiova with the diagnosis of anorexia nervosa, the patient

		lost 21 kg in 2 months.
2.		Current mental state:
	a)	General appearance: neat appearance, depressed face, easy crying, uncooperativeness, irritability
	b)	Behavior: denies the existence of problems, low tolerance for frustration
c)		Communication (speech/content): verbal contact is established with difficulty, but the patient states that she gets along well with other colleagues.
		Nonverbal: visual contact is easily made but not maintained, the gaze is directed downwards
	d)	Mood: isolated, withdrawn, sad mood
	e)	Orientation: temporal-spatial
	f)	Sleep: physiological

	d)	How the patient understands his illness: he denies the existence of some problems
	h)	The family's attitude towards the patient's illness: the patient is cared for by her grandmother who accompanies her, the mother is very worried about the girl's condition, she said that "she doesn't know what else to do to make her daughter feel better"

3. Subjects of concern for the patient:

- food refusal

- obsessive preoccupation with weight

- severe weight loss

V. Additional information:

The patient, aged 16 years and 7 months, student in the 8th grade, is hospitalized in the 5th ward of the Pr. Dr. Alexandru Obregia Hospital for:

- food refusal

- obsessive preoccupation with body weight

- distorted body image

The patient was hospitalized in the last two months in the Pediatric Craiova with the diagnosis of anorexia nervosa, severe malnutrition following food refusal, from where she was transferred to our clinic for the establishment of therapeutic behavior.

The patient comes accompanied by her grandmother to our ward for the reappearance of exaggerated weight concerns.

The patient associates the onset of symptoms with the critical statement from a colleague "she told me that I am fat and ugly and I need to lose weight"

The patient's parents are divorced, the patient does not keep in touch with her father, whom she only knows by sight.

Other data

Laboratory data

GLU – 78 mg/dl

TP – 6.1 g/dl

CA – 8.0 mg/dl

AST – 20 U/L

ALT – 19 U/L

Ca $^{2+}$ - 1.80 MEg/L

Thymol – 1UML

HGB – 13.9 g/dL

L – 10.9 10^6/μL

H – 4.5 10^6/μL

Hz – 37.8%

T – 26.1 10^3/μL

EEG:

The EEG trace with diffuse bioelectric changes and voltage with tendencies to flatten the background trace. Hyperventilation does not significantly change the long-distance route; without paroxysmal discharges.

Psychological examination:

Anxious experiences related to the possibility of getting fat, distorted image of the silhouette, intense preoccupations to lose weight, relational inadequacy, the accentuated need to receive affection, over-appreciation, self-idealization, act in an orderly, methodical manner.

It shows restlessness, instability, irritability.

Under treatment with Olanzapine 15mg/day; Thioridazine 150 mg/day; Zoloft 100 mg/day; polyvitamins 2 tb/ day; 6 Glubifer 3 tb/day, the clinical evolution is satisfactory.

He is discharged at the request of the family with the recommendation to continue the treatment.

C. Data analysis and interpretation

Anorexia is a very serious eating behavior disorder, without treatment it leads to the emergence of not easy complications and even death.

The nurse must be patient with the patient, understanding, calm and firm with the patient. She must give the patient and the family as many details as possible about the disease and its treatment.

Basically, anorexics refuse to admit that they have a disorder and oppose any intervention aimed at their eating behavior, but at the same time they can more easily accept help to solve other problems.

The nurse, together with the patient and his family, will draw up the care plan, establish the schedule and content of the meals, taking into account the patient's food preferences, and will use different therapy techniques.

In family therapy, the nurse has the role of:

- helps the family to express their needs

- helps the patient to modify and control her answers

- discuss difficult problems in the family

- actively participates in finding solutions without imposing a certain option.

D. CARE PLAN

PURPOSE – LONG TERM

Date	No. Fr.	Identified needs/problems (Dr. Nursing)	Desired result (goal - short term)	Interventions (Actions/Date/Time)	Signature	Result obtained
07.	1	Nutritio	The	- I established		

05.		nal	patient	together with the		
09		deficit,	will	patient and her		
		related	restore	grandmother the		
		to self-	her	schedule and		
		deprivati	normal	organization of		
		on of	body	meals, 4 small		
		food and	weight	portions per day.		
		hyperact		- I went with the		
		ivity		patient to the		
				dining room,		
				where she ate		
				with all the other		
				patients in my		
				presence.		
				- I supervised the		
				patient during		
				and after the		
				meal to avoid the		
				provocation of		
				vomiting and not		
				to throw away		
				the food.		
				- I congratulated		
				the patient when		

				she managed to eat everything we proposed - I talked with the grandmother saying that a visible progress was obtained in terms of nutrition and body weight - I weighed the patient daily, in the morning in the same outfit. - I tried by distracting the patient after each meal to make the patient stop crying by training her in different games in the playroom (card game, stick game)		

		2	Disturbance of self-esteem associated with a low tolerance to frustration, related to the need to please others, to be approved, accepted	The patient will show an increase in self-esteem, she will gain more confidence in her own strength	- I encouraged her to define her own interests (preferred activities) to make her feel less disinterested by gaining control over herself - I talked with the patient about what she likes to do, how she would like to be in relationships with her parents and others and how acceptance will be achieved. - I strengthened the patient's strengths, valued her by making her		

					more confident in her own strengths		
		3	Social isolation, disruption of interpersonal relationships due to the fear of being rejected.	The patient will relate more easily to others and participate in group activities or other social activities	- I helped the patient talk about her feelings of loneliness through permanent interactions with her several times a day. - I showed a sincere interest to the patient, trying to convince her that I care about her - I encourage the patient to look for ways to spend her free time, to be able to relax, to broaden her		

				social contacts. - I recommended the patient to avoid conflicts of any kind both with her grandmother and with her colleagues through tolerance and self-confidence.		
	4	Anxiety about gaining weight and losing control over food	The patient will talk more easily about her fears	- I encouraged the patient to talk about her fears, implicitly about gaining weight and losing control over food. - through systematic discussions every day, I explained to the patient		

				that there is progress in solving her major problems by gaining weight without distorting her image of her physique - I presented her with a table showing the ideal weight for her age and height - I discussed with the patient about the foods that do not pose a risk of making you fat, but on the contrary can be very beneficial in order to obtain a good functionality of		

				the body (e.g. fruits, vegetables, dairy products)		
	5	Disturbance of family dynamics due to rigidity in the exercise of roles	The family will become more understanding, will be more open to the patient's problems and will encourage her to act	- I evaluated family relationships - through discussions with the mother, different ways of approaching her relations with her daughter were suggested - from the dialogue with the patient's mother, she comes to the conclusion that she needs to reorganize her ideas and approach to situations. The		

| | | | autono mously | patient will be controlled by the mother "from the shadows" without emphasizing the idea of eating out of obligation, thus de-escalating the conflict between them
- finally, the family is willing to adopt an open dialogue between them based on sincerity, which will help them have a harmonious relationship with the family. | | |

E. ASSESSMENT AND THE PATIENT'S RESPONSE TO CARE

Da te	No . pb.		Signatur e
As a result of the care performed, the objectives were not achieved at all			
	1	The patient started to eat better, but the weight gain did not exceed 1 ½ during the 2-week hospitalization, still maintaining control over the quality and quantity of food	
	2	The patient expressed her feelings referring to her own person and understood the functions and needs of the body	
		The patient has more self-confidence and has found ways to be accepted by others, showing tolerance and self-confidence	
		The patient wants to change her behavior, shows interest in the proposed activities and easily verbalizes her feelings.	
		The fear of not gaining weight has decreased in intensity, but it still persists.	

The family showed understanding for the patient's problems in order to de-tension the situation in the family as much as possible, he will be permanently always by her side, without feeling constrained. Specifically, after the grandmother's departure from the hospital, the patient stayed with us for another week, during which she settled in better, was relaxed, more available in conversations, relating well with the salon colleagues with whom she ate together and played various games activities.

Under treatment with Olanzapine 15mg/day; Thioridazine 150 mg/day; Zoloft 100 mg/day; polyvitamins 2 tb/day; 6 Glubifer 3 tb/day, the clinical evolution is satisfactory.

He is discharged at the request of the family with the recommendation to continue the treatment.

F) Conclusions

Eating disorders (anorexia and bulimia nervosa) generally appear during puberty and adolescence against a background of increased psychological vulnerability, considering the increasingly demanding socio-cultural conditions, attention is directed towards the masses of young people to prevent the installation of these disorders.

For this, the care network in the community will have to be developed, the preparation of educational programs for teenagers, the development of relations with the educational institutions where the young people work.

Case 3

I. Anamnestic data

Name, Surname – VS

Date of birth –
10.09.1994

Address, Telephone –
Bucharest,

Marital status -
unmarried

Current occupation -
student

Studies - 8th grade

Allergies - food

II. self help	Independent	Need help	addicted
1. Mobility	Yes	-	-
2. Feeding	-	Yes	-
3. Hygiene	Yes	-	-
4. Dressed	Yes	-	-
5. The continent	Yes	-	-

III. Patient description

a) Eye color: green

b) Hair color: blond

c) Height: 1.64 m

d) Weight: 37 kg

e) Skin: white

f) Teeth: complete dentition

g) Vision: good

h) Manners: does not present

i) Speech: coherence

j) Physical deformities/posture: none

2. The name the patient preferred: Dany

3. Distinctive features

4. Previous occupation: student

5. Hobbies and interests: reading, listening to music

6. Family members or significant persons in the patient's life: maternal grandparents, maternal aunt and mother.

7. People who could visit him / Social support: grandparents, aunt (the patient is hospitalized with her mother.

8. Living conditions: she lives in a two-room apartment with her maternal grandparents, maternal aunt and mother (46 years old, no longer working for medical reasons, parents are divorced, the patient does not keep in touch with her father, whom she only knows from view.)

IV. Mental condition

1	Previous mental illnesses: The patient was hospitalized in the pediatric hospital in Craiova with the diagnosis of anorexia nervosa, the patient lost 21 kg in 2 months.
2.	Current mental state:
	a) General appearance: neat appearance, depressed face, easy crying, uncooperativeness, irritability
	b) Behavior: denies the existence of problems, low tolerance for frustration
c)	Communication (speech/content): verbal contact is established with difficulty, but the

		patient states that she gets along well with other colleagues.
		Nonverbal: visual contact is easily made but not maintained, the gaze is directed downwards
	d)	Mood: isolated, withdrawn, sad mood
	e)	Orientation: temporal-spatial
	f)	Sleep: physiological
	d)	How the patient understands his illness: he denies the existence of some problems
	h)	The family's attitude towards the patient's illness: the patient is cared for by her grandmother who accompanies her, the mother is very worried about the girl's condition, she said that "she doesn't know what else to do to make her daughter feel better"

3. Subjects of concern for the patient:

- food refusal

- obsessive preoccupation with weight

- severe weight loss

V. Additional information:

The patient, aged 15 years and 7 months, student in the 8th grade, is hospitalized in the 5th ward of the Pr. Dr. Alexandru Obregia Hospital for:

- food refusal

- obsessive preoccupation with body weight

- distorted body image

The patient was hospitalized in the last two months in the Pediatric Hospital in Craiova with the diagnosis of anorexia nervosa, severe malnutrition following food refusal, from where she was transferred to our clinic for the establishment of therapeutic behavior.

The patient comes accompanied by her grandmother to our ward for the reappearance of exaggerated weight concerns.

The patient associates the onset of symptoms with the critical statement from a colleague "she told me that I am fat and ugly and I need to lose weight"

The patient's parents are divorced, the patient does not keep in touch with her father, whom she only knows by sight.

Other data

Laboratory data

GLU – 78 mg/dl

TP – 6.1 g/dl

CA – 8.0 mg/dl

AST – 20 U/L

ALT – 19 U/L

Ca^{2+} - 1.80 MEg/L

Thymol – 1UML

HGB – 13.9 g/dL

L – 10.9 10^6/µL

H – 4.5 10^6/µL

Hz – 37.8%

T – 26.1 10^3/µL

EEG:

The EEG trace with diffuse bioelectric changes and voltage with tendencies to flatten the background trace.

Hyperventilation does not significantly change the long-distance route; without paroxysmal discharges.

Psychological examination:

Anxious experiences related to the possibility of getting fat, distorted image of the silhouette, intense preoccupations to lose weight, relational inadequacy, the accentuated need to receive affection, over-appreciation, self-idealization, act in an orderly, methodical manner.

It shows restlessness, instability, irritability.

Under treatment with Olanzapine 15mg/day; Thioridazine 150 mg/day; Zoloft 100 mg/day; polyvitamins 2 tb/ day; 6 Glubifer 3 tb/day, the clinical evolution is satisfactory.

He is discharged at the request of the family with the recommendation to continue the treatment.

C. Data analysis and interpretation

Anorexia is a very serious eating behavior disorder, without treatment it leads to the emergence of not easy complications and even death.

The nurse must be patient with the patient, understanding, calm and firm with the patient. She must give the patient and the family as many details as possible about the disease and its treatment.

Basically, anorexics refuse to admit that they have a disorder and oppose any intervention aimed at their eating behavior, but at the same time they can more easily accept help to solve other problems.

The nurse, together with the patient and his family, will draw up the care plan, establish the schedule and content of the meals, taking into account the patient's food preferences, and will use different therapy techniques.

In family therapy, the nurse has the role of:

- helps the family to express their needs

- helps the patient to modify and control her answers

- discuss difficult problems in the family

- actively participates in finding solutions without imposing a certain option.

D. CARE PLAN

PURPOSE – LONG TERM

Date	No. Fr.	Identified needs/problems (Dr. Nursing)	Desired result (goal - short term)	Interventions (Actions/Date/Time)	Signature	Result obtained
07. 05. 09	1	Nutritional deficit, related to self-deprivation of food and hyperactivity	The patient will restore her normal body weight	- I established together with the patient and her grandmother the schedule and organization of meals, 4 small portions per day. - I went with the patient to the dining room, where she ate with all the other patients in my presence. - I supervised the		

				patient during and after the meal to avoid the provocation of vomiting and not to throw away the food. - I congratulated the patient when she managed to eat everything we proposed - I talked with the grandmother saying that a visible progress was obtained in terms of nutrition and body weight - I weighed the patient daily, in the morning in the same outfit. - I tried by		

				distracting the patient after each meal to make the patient stop crying by training her in different games in the playroom (card game, stick game)		
	2	Disturbance of self-esteem associated with a low tolerance to frustration, related to the need to	The patient will show an increase in self-esteem, she will gain more confid	- I encouraged her to define her own interests (preferred activities) to make her feel less disinterested by gaining control over herself - I talked with the patient about what she likes to do, how she would like to be		

| | | please others, to be approved, accepted | ence in her own strength | in relationships with her parents and others and how acceptance will be achieved. - I strengthened the patient's strengths, valued her by making her more confident in her own strengths | | |
| | 3 | Social isolation, disruption of interpersonal relationships due to the fear of being | The patient will relate more easily to others and participate in group | - I helped the patient talk about her feelings of loneliness through permanent interactions with her several times a day. - I showed a sincere interest to the patient, | | |

		rejected.	activities or other social activities	trying to convince her that I care about her - I encourage the patient to look for ways to spend her free time, to be able to relax, to broaden her social contacts. - I recommended the patient to avoid conflicts of any kind both with her grandmother and with her colleagues through tolerance and self-confidence.		
	4	Anxiety about gaining	The patient will	- I encouraged the patient to talk about her fears,		

		weight and losing control over food	talk more easily about her fears	implicitly about gaining weight and losing control over food. - through systematic discussions every day, I explained to the patient that there is progress in solving her major problems by gaining weight without distorting her image of her physique - I presented her with a table showing the ideal weight for her age and height - I discussed with the patient about		

| | | | | the foods that do not pose a risk of making you fat, but on the contrary can be very beneficial in order to obtain a good functionality of the body (e.g. fruits, vegetables, dairy products) | | |
| | 5 | Disturbance of family dynamics due to rigidity in the exercise of roles | The family will become more understanding, will be more open to the | - I evaluated family relationships
- through discussions with the mother, different ways of approaching her relations with her daughter were suggested
- from the | | |

			patient's problems and will encourage her to act autonomously	dialogue with the patient's mother, she comes to the conclusion that she needs to reorganize her ideas and approach to situations. The patient will be controlled by the mother "from the shadows" without emphasizing the idea of eating out of obligation, thus de-escalating the conflict between them - finally, the family is willing to adopt an open dialogue between		

| | | | them based on sincerity, which will help them have a harmonious relationship with the family. | | |

E. ASSESSMENT AND THE PATIENT'S RESPONSE TO CARE

Date	No. pb.		Signature
As a result of the care performed, the objectives were not achieved at all			
	1	The patient started to eat better, but the weight gain did not exceed 1 ½ during the 2-week hospitalization, still maintaining control over the quality and quantity of food	
	2	The patient expressed her feelings referring to her own person and understood the functions and needs of the body	

		The patient has more self-confidence and has found ways to be accepted by others, showing tolerance and self-confidence	
		The patient wants to change her behavior, shows interest in the proposed activities and easily verbalizes her feelings.	
		The fear of not gaining weight has decreased in intensity, but it still persists.	
		The family showed understanding for the patient's problems in order to de-tension the situation in the family as much as possible, he will be permanently always by her side, without feeling constrained. Specifically, after the grandmother's departure from the hospital, the patient stayed with us for another week, during which she settled in better, was relaxed, more available in conversations, relating well with the salon colleagues with whom she ate together and played various games activities. Under treatment with Olanzapine	

		15mg/day; Thioridazine 150 mg/day; Zoloft 100 mg/day; polyvitamins 2 tb/day; 6 Glubifer 3 tb/day, the clinical evolution is satisfactory. He is discharged at the request of the family with the recommendation to continue the treatment.	

F) Conclusions

Eating disorders (anorexia and bulimia nervosa) generally appear during puberty and adolescence against a background of increased psychological vulnerability, considering the increasingly demanding socio-cultural conditions, attention is directed towards the masses of young people to prevent the installation of these disorders.

For this, the care network in the community will have to be developed, the preparation of educational programs for teenagers, the development of relations with the educational institutions where the young people work. It is necessary to develop educational programs regarding eating disorders among young people, since they have a psychiatric and not an organic origin. It is desirable for the adolescent to know and understand his role in society.

Selective Bibliography

- Small encyclopedic atlas-Ana Bogdan, Septimiu Chelcea

 - *Dictionary of social psychology*-Prof. Dr. Petru Meila, Prof. Dr. Stefan Milea – *Treatise on paediatrics*

-Dr. Maria Georgescu – *Practical guide*

-Prof. Dr. Constantin Enachescu – *Treatise on mental hygiene*

-Dr. Ileana Raut - *Psychiatry course*

-I would. Fr. Mariana Federiga – *Nursing models*

-Barbara Flynn Sideleanu – *Psychiatric Nursing*

- Murariu Letitia, Ivan Mariuca, Puiu Victoria, Spataru Ruxandra, Tofan Ruxandra, Chiru Florian, Stoianovici Serban - *Theoretical and practical bases of caring for healthy and sick people.*